GRAVES DISEASE NATURAL HEALING

By Smith J. Offor

Table of Contents

Introduction

Natural Treatment Options for Graves' Disease

An autoimmune condition called Graves' disease causes hyperthyroidism. Writing a number of web pages on hypothyroidism helped me get my first job working with Graves' disease patients. I wrote a few paragraphs about Graves' disease without giving it much thought. As it turned out, there is so little information available on Graves' disease that this was all it took to get patients calling my office.

It's unfortunate that there isn't more information about Graves' disease in the natural health community because there are effective natural treatments available.

Generally speaking, it's critical to treat the person, not the illness.

Generally speaking, the priority should be on the individual rather than the disease.

It's usually important to treat the individual, not the disease.

As a rule, the priority should be on the individual rather than the disease.

The main focus is on treating the individual, not diagnosing the illness.

In general, it's important to treat the person, not disease.

The practitioner must be knowledgeable about standard therapies, methods for diagnosing illnesses, and supplements and medications that are used to manage symptoms.

that having Graves' disease is always an emergency.

Even though it's rare, Graves' disease can occasionally worsen into a thyroid storm that could be fatal. Thyroid storm affects approximately 0.22 percent of all patients with thyrotoxic disease, according to a study of the condition's prevalence in Japan. 2 Patients who have not been taking their medications as prescribed frequently experience this.

The typical Graves disease presentation

The following are the most typical signs of hyperthyroidism that my patients with Graves' disease present with:

- elevated heart rate.

- Palpitations.

- Hypertension.

- Anxiety.

- tremors in the muscles.

- intolerance to heat.

- loss of weight

- Goiter

- Dry, hot skin and a long, bloody tongue.

- increased bowel movement.

About 3% of patients with Graves' disease experience Graves' dermopathy (pretibial myxedema).

In 20 to 40 percent of cases, Graves' ophthalmopathy is noticeable. One in five to ten patients will experience severe lymphocytic infiltration of the eye muscles, which will cause the eye to protrude. Patients occasionally have Graves' ophthalmopathy without being hyperthyroid.

When thyroid hormone levels are normal but thyroid-stimulating hormone (TSH) is low, subclinical hyperthyroidism is present. Subclinical hyperthyroidism can last for many years and does not always develop into overt hyperthyroidism

Some people will experience all of the typical symptoms mentioned above. Others, though, will only have a few. A wide range of symptoms, from the barely perceptible to fatal, can be associated with hyperthyroidism.

Patients may experience emotional symptoms that can be associated with bipolar disorder or anxiety. It is possible for mental symptoms to come on first.

It's critical to understand that not every person with hyperthyroidism will present in the same way in order to avoid misdiagnoses. Don't assume someone doesn't have hyperthyroidism just because they don't fit the stereotype.

Test for diagnosis
TSH, thyroxine (T4), triiodothyronine (T3), and a complete blood count should be included in the initial blood workup for Graves' disease. A group of antibodies that cause hyperthyroidism are detected using the TSI (thyroid-stimulating immunoglobulins) test. Ninety percent of

Graves' disease patients have positive test results. Antibodies to thyroid peroxidase (TPO) and thyroglobulin (TG) are frequently found as well.

Other laboratory tests may change as a result of hyperthyroidism. For instance, you might notice increased glucose and liver enzymes.

Using a radioactive uptake scan, Graves' disease is frequently identified. Due to this, Graves' disease can be distinguished from other hyperthyroidism-causing conditions.

Radioactive iodine uptake scans are frequently recommended by endocrinologists to their patients. Many patients are worried about possible risks associated with this test.

Patients' worries and customary treatments

Even in cases where symptoms are mild, endocrinologists frequently advise radioactive iodine therapy (RAI) to kill the thyroid gland. It's important to be able to talk with patients about the negative effects of RAI if they come to you for a second opinion because endocrinologists may not always educate their patients about these effects.

Several things about RAI to be aware of

Even after RAI, some people will still have Graves' disease because RAI is not always effective.

15% of patients seem to have worsening Graves' ophthalmopathy3.

After RAI, a lot of patients simply don't feel well, or other medical issues could develop.

Only after reading numerous unfavorable, anecdotal stories online may patients decide to visit a naturopathic physician.

Unsurprisingly, an autoimmune condition like Graves' disease is not a random occurrence.

The Graves' disease's underlying causes won't be addressed in any way by RAI; they will continue to exist.

The most frequently prescribed drug for symptom control is methimazole. Women who are pregnant or nursing are administered propylthiouracil (since methimazole is not advised in these circumstances). Both of these drugs come with a long list of harmful side effects, including pruritus, allergic dermatitis, nausea, and dyspepsia. Agranulocytosis is a severe side effect, though it is rare, and it usually shows up within the first 60 days of starting a medication.

Blood pressure medication like propranolol is frequently prescribed for this purpose.

When beginning a natural protocol, patients frequently wonder if they must stop taking their medications. I assure them that doing both at once is acceptable. As they recover, they can talk to their endocrinologist about reducing their medication dosage.

Reaching the Cause

There is no one protocol that works for all patients with Graves' disease.

Everybody is unique.

Simply put, you should think about the following.

Autoimmune disease and a compromised digestive system are frequently linked. It has been hypothesized that Yersinia enterocolitica may be the cause of Graves' disease. There might also be a connection between Helicobacter pylori and Graves' disease.

Especially with gluten, think about food allergies. 9 Inquire of patients whether they use artificial sweeteners, which there is anecdotal evidence may contribute to hyperthyroidism.

toxicology and lymphatic stagnation. I obtain a thorough history of any injuries that might be connected to the region around the thyroid. This covers any prior head or neck injuries, dental work, tonsillitis, respiratory infections, ear or sinus infections, or dental work. Around the neck, look for swollen lymph nodes. Are their tonsils still present?

Natural Medicine for Symptom Control

Hydrotherapy and herbs that stimulate the lymphatic system, like Trifoliumpratense, are just two of the treatments available to improve blood and lymphatic circulation. I believe it is preferable to simply take a full history and treat the patient as a whole rather than automatically choosing a lymphatic herb from a predetermined list to treat hyperthyroidism.

Biotherapeutic drainage is one main treatment methods.

With this detoxification system, toxins that have been stored in the body are released, and symptoms are controlled by the use of compound homeopathics. In many cases, these are combined with isopathic medicines.

You can manage Graves' disease symptoms by taking the following supplements. A natural treatment strategy, though, should go further and try to address the underlying cause rather than stopping here.

Lithium

It is well known that lithium carbonate on prescription can result in hypothyroidism. Lithium carbonate is effective at reducing the symptoms of hyperthyroidism, according to small studies. There are also case reports of patients who received a lithium prescription for another reason but later developed Graves' disease and remained asymptomatic while taking lithium.

Due to the toxicity of lithium carbonate prescribed by a doctor, conventional medicine does not recommend lithium for the treatment of hyperthyroidism.

However, low-dose lithium orotate is offered by a number of businesses; it typically contains 5 mg per capsule. I take a medication that contains 150 mcg of lithium per tablet (derived from a vegetable culture), dosed at 1-3 tablets TID depending on the severity of my symptoms.

Although I'm not aware of any, it would be beneficial to have clinical studies on the efficacy of nutritional lithium for hyperthyroidism. Through the advice of the company I use, I learned about using lithium. On his website, Jonathan Wright has a well-written article about the benefits and security of lithium. I tried lithium with my clients after being unsatisfied with the efficacy of other hyperthyroidism supplements and discovered that it works incredibly well in Graves' disease.

I did have one case of hyperthyroidism brought on by a thyroid nodule, and lithium had absolutely no effect on her; she had to return to the doctors.

Selenium

For treating Graves' disease symptoms, including ophthalmopathy, a daily dose of 200 mcg has been found to be effective.

Carnitine

In the scientific literature, it has been demonstrated that L-carnitine, dosed at 2 or 4 g per day, improves hyperthyroidism symptoms. But if lithium and sedative herbs work, patients might not need to spend extra money on supplements.

Herbs

Herbs used for anxiety or to calm the heart are frequently prescribed for hyperthyroidism.

The most famous of these is Lycopusvirginicus. Traditional treatments for hyperthyroidism also included the use of melissaofficinalis, leonuruscardiaca, and other calming herbs.

Iodine: What Is It?

There are numerous alternative supplements that can be used safely and effectively; I don't see any benefit in using iodine when it may possibly worsen symptoms. Iodine supplementation after remission may increase the risk of recurrence, according to studies.

Medications:

- 5 mg/day of methimazole.

First Protocol:

- 50 mcg TID of lithium orotate.

- 100 mcg/day of selenium.

- Avoid sugar, dairy, and gluten.

- Less dry skin than before.

- The bleeding is now less easy.

As an alternative, the thyroid should simply stop making extra thyroid hormone. Due to this, some people can have very low TSH levels while still having no symptoms and normal levels of thyroid hormones.

Although it was explained to her that this was just an initial protocol meant to control symptoms and that more work needed to be done, the mother turned down a more extensive supplement protocol due to financial constraints. They still come by to pick up more lithium even though there haven't been any follow-up visits since then. Lithium should ideally only be used to treat symptoms while addressing the underlying immune system triggers. The patient would be better off, in my opinion, on a small dose of nutritional lithium than on a dangerous pharmaceutical that wasn't even that effective at controlling symptoms.

Isopathic medicines, created in accordance with the Enderlein philosophy, are an effective way to control immune response. Although they don't directly affect the body, they will still cause a strong immune response because they are made from non-viable fungi or bacteria. They can be very beneficial in immune system-related conditions like autoimmune disease and chronic infections. The first product's primary effect was to reduce inflammation while inducing the immune system to eliminate an infection that hadn't been fully resolved. The other products function similarly but target infections more specifically. For a synergistic result, they can be combined.

To regulate thyroid function, balance minerals, improve liver and kidney function, and aid lymphatic drainage, various compound homeopathics were administered; each dose was 14 tsp BID. Opening up routes of elimination and preventing a potential harsh detoxification response from the isopathic remedies were the main goals of these homeopathics.

Additionally, a functional stool test was requested.

One-Month Follow-up:

- Overall, the patient is feeling much better.
- At 108/70 mmHg, blood pressure is now considered normal.
- 80 beats per minute.

- a sore throat. This was interpreted as a positive sign and likely a detoxification response from the isopathics.

5 Reasons for Graves' Disease and 5 Treatments

An overactive thyroid, also known as hyperthyroidism, is thought to affect between 3 and 10 million people. 1 Graves' disease is an autoimmune condition and is the most typical type of hyperthyroidism.

Describe Graves' disease

Your thyroid, a butterfly-shaped gland in the front of your neck, creates hormones that help control things like body temperature, heart rate, growth, and the health of your brain. When the thyroid produces too much thyroid hormone, hyperthyroidism develops. A body will burn through nutrients too quickly if its thyroid hormone levels are too high, which will speed up its energy metabolism.

Malnutrition and chronic diseases may follow from this. I ate everything in sight as I battled Graves' disease, going from a size 4 to a size 0 in a matter of months.

The autoimmune condition is frequently to blame for the overactive thyroid, though there are other causes as well. 60 to 80 percent of cases of hyperthyroidism are caused by Graves' disease. Normally, the pituitary gland, a tiny organ that secretes the thyroid stimulating hormone (TSH), which instructs the thyroid to produce the thyroid hormones T3 and T4, controls thyroid function. Thyrotropin receptor antibody (TRAb) is an antibody that can mimic pituitary hormones in Graves' disease and completely override the system, causing an overactive thyroid.

Anti-thyroglobulin antibodies as well as antibodies against thyroid peroxidase (TPO) can form.

Toxic multinodular goiter and toxic adenoma are two additional types of hyperthyroidism that aren't caused by autoimmune diseases. On the thyroid gland itself, toxic multinodular goiter is characterized by the development of nodules that can function independently. Without the aid of TSH, these nodules can stimulate the thyroid, disrupting the production of thyroid hormones and leading to an overactive thyroid.

Thyroid follicular cells that overproduce T3 and/or T4 make up the benign tumor known as a toxic adenoma. Hyperthyroidism can result from toxic adenomas' overproduction of thyroid hormones, which can inhibit the function of the thyroid's remaining healthy tissue.

<

Symptoms of Graves' disease

- A hot flash and sweating
- unintentional loss of weight.
- diarrhea or stools that are frequently loose.
- insomnia and a hard time falling asleep.
- constant fatigue, irritability, or anxiety.
- increased heart rate.
- modifications to menstrual cycles.
- lower libido.
- eyes that bulge.
- thick red skin on the feet or shins.
- an increase in appetite.
- Osteoporosis.

- shaky hands.

- muscular lassitude.

The method for diagnosing Graves' disease

1. The initial step is to have your thyroid hormone levels checked via blood tests. TSH will be extremely low and the levels of free T4 and free T3 will be elevated in hyperthyroidism. Antibody levels will also be increased in autoimmune diseases.

2. The next stage in the diagnosis of a thyroid imbalance is radioactive iodine uptake (RAIU). The amount of iodine the thyroid absorbs will be determined by an RAIU using a low dose of I-131. The presence of Graves' disease is indicated by a high iodine uptake. This examination can

be useful in excluding other thyroid overactivity-related causes.

3. To examine thyroid nodules, thyroid ultrasound (US) is a useful procedure. To confirm that the nodules are not cancerous, your doctor might ask you to undergo a fine needle biopsy.

Hyperthyroidism's causes

1. Gluten

Worse yet, gluten can cause havoc on your gut and set you up for a leaky gut due to its hybridization and modification, its widespread consumption, and its many health risks. Gluten can enter the bloodstream once the gut is damaged, confusing the immune system. Because your thyroid gland and gluten have similar molecular compositions, a process known as molecular mimicry—where the immune system mistakenly attacks your own cells— can occur.

2. Gut leakage

The gut is somewhat permeable to extremely small molecules, which allows it to absorb nutrients. Numerous factors, such as gluten, infections, medications, and stress, can harm the gut, allowing toxins, microbes, and undigested food particles to enter the bloodstream unfiltered. Leaky gut is the entry point for infections, toxins, and inflammatory food particles to cause systemic inflammation and autoimmune disease. Before you can reverse uncomfortable symptoms, your gut needs to be repaired.

3. Mercury

The cells of various bodily tissues can be altered or harmed by the heavy metal mercury. When damaged cells are mistaken for foreign invaders, your immune system may start attacking your organs. According to studies, those who are exposed to more mercury have a higher risk of developing autoimmune thyroid disease.

4. Infections

Through inflammation and molecular mimicry, infections like the Epstein-Barr virus (EBV) and the herpes family of viruses (HSV) have been suggested as potential causes of autoimmune thyroid disease.

5. Iodine

The status of iodine is somewhat debatable. It appears that iodine levels that are too low or too high can lead to goiter and hypothyroidism, respectively. The thyroid may start producing more thyroid hormone when the body senses that there is more iodine available. If a person with a relatively low iodine intake abruptly switches to a very high-iodine diet, over time, that person may produce an excessive amount of thyroid hormone, leading to an overactive thyroid.

Graves' disease conventional treatment

Conventional medicine only focuses on treating symptoms; it doesn't address the underlying causes of the disease. Surgery, radiation, and medications only address the overactive thyroid gland in an effort to lessen disease symptoms. I advise using a functional medicine strategy to help identify the root cause of the imbalance in order to effectively treat the condition and repair your thyroid and immune system. My biggest regret in life stems from my personal attempts at two of these three conventional treatments.

1. Medications

An antithyroid medication called propylthiouracil (PTU) prevents the thyroid hormones from being produced.

You can find a long list of harmful side effects for these medications by searching online, one of which is liver damage.

Another anti-thyroid medication used to treat hyperthyroidism is methimazole. The TSH and Free T4 levels need to be carefully monitored because this medication can actually cause hypothyroidism. Aplastic anemia, rash, hair loss, vertigo, jaundice, lupus-like syndrome, and hepatitis are just a few of the side effects.

2. Radiation/Ablation

With this method, thyroid gland cells are fatally damaged using a large dose of radioactive iodine (I-131). You will need to take thyroid hormone medication for the rest of your life after this procedure. There was no other option after contracting toxic hepatitis from the PTU than to administer my own treatment. As I have done with many patients in my clinic

3. Surgery

Doctors may advise a partial thyroidectomy, which is when part of the thyroid gland is surgically removed, when antithyroid drugs and radioactive treatments are not practical alternatives. If a person is unable to reverse their hyperthyroidism using a functional medicine approach, it is advised to try this option as a last resort.

Graves' Disease: A Functional Medicine Approach

Instead of just treating the symptoms or turning to drastic measures, treating the underlying causes of your hyperthyroidism head-on is the key to reversing Graves' disease. The Myers Way 30-day plan is the method used to describe in detail how to do this.The Thyroid Connection.The fundamental of this strategy is shown below:

1. Cut gluten out of your diet

Because gluten is an inflammatory food, I advise all of my patients to cut it out of their diets. I strongly advise patients with autoimmune conditions like Graves' or Hashimoto's thyroiditis to cut out all grains and legumes from their diets. These foods contain lectins, proteins that damage the lining of your gut and serve as a natural pesticide for crops. The first step to recovery is a diet change.

2. Rebuild Your Gut

You must repair your gut in order to heal yourself. The exact same procedures used with patients to help repair leaky gut are outlined in the Myers Way Leaky Gut Breakthrough Program.

3. Perform a heavy metals test

A number of factors can expose us to heavy metals, including amalgam fillings, eating fish, and the environment. If you want to find out if mercury or other heavy metals are a problem for you, Its advised having your MTHFR genes tested and taking a DMPS chelation challenge test through a functional medicine practitioner.

4. Locate and treat infections

Have your doctor perform tests for HSV and EBV infections. It has been demonstrated that adding monolaurin from coconut oil to treatments for both HSV and EBV can be very beneficial. In order to fight HSV infections, a lysine-rich diet is also helpful.

5. Take Care of Your Immune System

Strong immune modulators, such as vitamin D, omega-3 fish oils, and glutathione, can support your immune system. It has been demonstrated that vitamin D aids in immune system regulation. Omega 3 fish oils aid in the body's overall fight against inflammation. The most potent antioxidant in your body,

glutathione, can lessen inflammation and
enhance detoxification pathways.

Thyroid hyperfunction and Graves' disease

When the thyroid gland produces too much thyroid hormone, it is called hyperthyroidism. About 1% of all Americans have this disorder, and women are much more likely to be affected than men. In its mildest form, hyperthyroidism may not manifest any symptoms; however, in some patients, an excess of thyroid hormone and its effects on the body may have serious repercussions.

The causes of hyperthyroidism

Hyperthyroidism can be caused by a number of things:

One toxic nodule or lump in the thyroid can cause hyperthyroidism by producing more thyroid hormone than the body requires.

Toxic multinodular goiter: If the thyroid gland has multiple nodules, sometimes those nodules can produce too much thyroid hormone, which can lead to hyperthyroidism. Patients over 50 are the ones who experience this the most frequently. A multinodular goiter frequently takes years to begin producing too much thyroid hormone in the body of the patient.

An autoimmune disorder called Graves' disease causes the thyroid to be attacked by the body's immune system. The thyroid gland enlarges and frequently becomes hyperthyroid in Graves' disease patients. The eyes of some patients may be impacted. Patients might experience double vision, a gritty sensation, general eye irritation, increased tear production, or their eyes become more prominent. They might also notice that their eyelids do not close completely. This condition is much more common in women than in men and, like other autoimmune diseases, may affect other family members.

Subacute thyroiditis is a form of hyperthyroidism that can occur after a viral infection that inflames the thyroid gland. Hyperthyroidism results from the thyroid's overproduction of thyroid hormone as a result of the inflammation. The thyroid usually returns to normal over time. Due to the release of the stored thyroid hormone, patients may experience hypothyroidism (where the thyroid gland produces insufficient thyroid hormone) for a while before the thyroid gland can restock its stores of thyroid hormone.

One to two months after giving birth, some women experience postpartum thyroiditis, which is characterized by mild to moderate hyperthyroidism. Hypothyroidism frequently follows this for several months. The majority of women heal and have healthy thyroid function.

Consuming too much iodine - Patients may occasionally develop hyperthyroidism as a result of consuming foods high in iodine, such as x-ray dyes, kelp tablets, some expectorants, over-the-counter supplements, and amiodarone (a medication used to treat certain heart rhythm issues). The hyperthyroidism typically goes away once the supplement is stopped.

Thyroid hormone overdose - Patients who take excessive amounts of thyroid hormone replacement may also develop hyperthyroidism. Patients should NEVER self-administer "extra" doses of thyroid hormone unless specifically instructed to do so by a doctor. Instead, they should have their thyroid hormone levels checked by a doctor at least once a year. Thyroid function testing should always be used as a guide when changing thyroid medication.

Hyperthyroidism signs and symptoms

- heartbeat that is erratic or rapid.

- agitation or anxiety.

- shaking of the hands.

- even though they ate as much as they normally would, they lost weight.

- sweating more and having hot flashes.

- hair loss on the scalp.
- separation of the nail bed from the fingernails.
- muscle wasting, especially in the thighs and upper arms.
- frequently having loose or irregular stools.
- skin alterations.
- a mysterious modification to women's menstrual cycles.
- an elevated risk of miscarriage.
- palpitations or a erratic heartbeat.
- bone density is reduced as a result of calcium loss from the bones.

How Is Hyperthyroidism Diagnosis Made?

Having hyperthyroidism has telltale signs and symptoms that a doctor can spot.

The signs and symptoms of hyperthyroidism are frequently vague and can be brought on by a wide variety of other conditions. The hyperthyroidism diagnosis and likely cause are verified through laboratory tests. The diagnosis of hyperthyroidism may be made by a primary care physician, but an endocrinologist—a doctor who specializes in thyroid and other endocrine diseases—might be required for assistance.

The thyroid stimulating hormone (TSH) level is the best test to determine overall thyroid function. To encourage the thyroid to produce and release more thyroid hormone, TSH is produced in the brain and moves to the thyroid gland. Thyroid hormone deficiency is indicated by a high TSH level. When the TSH level is below normal, it may be a sign of hyperthyroidism because the body typically produces more thyroid hormone than is needed. Free thyroxine (T4) and free triiodothyronine (T3) levels increase above normal when hyperthyroidism develops. Finding the cause of hyperthyroidism may be aided by additional laboratory investigations. When Graves' disease is the root cause of hyperthyroidism, TSIs (thyroid-stimulating immunoglobulins) can be found in the blood. Some diseases that result in hyperthyroidism also show thyroid peroxidase antibodies and other anti-thyroid antibodies.

Hyperthyroidism treatments

Depending on the cause, severity, and a number of other factors, there are currently a number of efficient treatments for hyperthyroidism. Antithyroid drugs, radioactive iodine, and thyroid surgery are the three most popular ways to treat hyperthyroidism.

Thyroid hormone production is lowered by antithyroid drugs, most frequently methimazole.

Antithyroid medication works while the patient is taking it but does not cure the disease. While in some patients the hyperthyroidism does go into remission and the medication can be stopped, it is not typically advised as a long-term solution. Thyroidectomy or radioactive iodine are frequently advised as more conclusive treatments if the hyperthyroidism does not go into remission after two years.

Hyperthyroidism is frequently treated with radioactive iodine (RAI).

Only a few body organs actively absorb iodine, including the thyroid.

As a result, the thyroid gland can be specifically damaged by radioactive iodine without affecting other organs. The body stops producing thyroid hormone when the thyroid gland eventually becomes destroyed and disappears. Patients with Graves' disease or those who have thyroid nodules causing hyperthyroidism can generally use this treatment.

Radioactive iodine doesn't always work well for treating hyperthyroidism.

Most patients will need levothyroxine (brand names Synthroid, Levothroid, and others) to replace their thyroid hormone after radioactive iodine. Once the proper thyroid hormone dosage for the patient has been established, thyroid hormone levels are frequently only checked once a year rather than frequently at first.

Some patients will undergo partial or complete thyroid removal surgery to treat their hyperthyroidism.

On a case-by-case basis, based on each patient's unique medical, social, and family history, it is decided which treatment for hyperthyroidism is the best treatment. In the following situations, surgical thyroidectomy is frequently advised over RAI.

RAI is unlikely to be an effective treatment for a large thyroid causing compressive symptoms.

Symptoms of compression and significant compression of nearby structures

Graves' eye disease that ranges from mild to severe.

- a failed medical treatment.

- adverse reaction to thyroid hormone-blocking drugs.

- Hyperthyroidism needs to be reversed quickly.

- Fear of radiation exposure and incapacity to follow radiation safety recommendations.

- thyroid nodules present simultaneously and thyroid cancer must be ruled out.

- at home with young children.

- pregnancy, desire to become pregnant within the next 4-6 months, or nursing.
- eagerness over time.

Our group of ophthalmologists specializes in treating Graves' disease, which can be difficult to manage. Treating patients with Graves' disease and Graves' eye disease is a challenge for the majority of ophthalmologists. If Graves' eye disease and hyperthyroidism co-occur in a patient, the severity of the eye disease will determine the type of hyperthyroidism treatment to be used.

While patients with mild or no Graves' eye disease may be candidates for any of the three hyperthyroidism treatment options, those with moderate to severe eye disease are frequently referred for surgical thyroidectomy because RAI has a higher risk of making the eye disease worse than surgery does.

Supporting Graves' Ophthalmopathy Treatments

An overactive thyroid gland is a hallmark of the autoimmune condition known as Graves' disease. Because of having too much thyroid hormone, it is the main cause of hyperthyroidism.

Graves' disease causes eye issues1 like swelling, redness, and, in some cases, vision loss in about 40% of patients who are diagnosed with it.

Graves' ophthalmopathy or thyroid eye disease is the medical name for this condition. The tissues around the eyes become inflamed as a result, probably as a result of the immune system mistakenly attacking these tissues.

Most people only experience mild Graves' ophthalmopathy, which may benefit from supportive or natural therapies until the condition gets better on its own over time. However, in a few instances, more severe symptoms appear, which frequently necessitate surgery.

Graves' disease symptoms in the eyes

The majority of Graves' disease patients only experience mild eye symptoms, such as redness, dryness, gritty eyes, sensitivity to light, and pain when moving their eyes.

However, one in ten people will experience more severe symptoms, such as:

- eyes that bulge or protrude due to severe eyelid swelling.
- When the eyes are not aligned properly, double vision results.
- optical nerve injury.
- blindness or a loss of vision.

Treatments that are conventional for Graves' ophthalmopathy

Steroids are the first line of treatment for mild to moderate Graves' ophthalmopathy in order to lessen swelling of the eye-area tissues.

If the steroids are ineffective, radiotherapy may be added to this. Both have side effects that you should discuss with your doctor.

It is now more common to use biological agents like Teprotumumab. Surgery is frequently required for eye diseases that pose a threat to vision.

Treatment options for Graves' ophthalmopathy

Within six months, the condition of about two-thirds of mild Graves' ophthalmopathy patients improves on its own. 2 Mild disease is frequently observed, and supportive therapy is typically all that is needed.

The condition is treated with the following supportive measures:

1. **supplementing the diet with selenium**

If you should try a selenium supplement, think about asking your doctor. A trace element called selenium can be found in foods like nuts, fish, beef, and grains as well as in water and soil. .

According to one European study, taking 100 g of selenium supplements twice a day slowed the progression of the disease3 and enhanced eye movements.

Although it is believed that European soil contains little selenium, it is unclear whether these European patients had low baseline blood selenium levels to begin with.

More research is required to determine whether selenium, which is present in our soil and may benefit American patients, may have any such benefits.

Additionally, it is still unclear how selenium might be able to lessen the signs and symptoms of Graves' ophthalmopathy.

Selenium must be used with caution because it can become toxic at high doses and cause adverse reactions like fatigue, nauseousness, diarrhea, and joint pain.

2. Exercising vitamin D

The study of vitamin D and Graves' ophthalmopathy4 is still being conducted. According to the most recent research, individuals with Graves' disease who are vitamin D deficient5 are more likely than those with normal vitamin D levels to develop Graves' eye disease.

The risk of developing Graves' ophthalmopathy and ongoing eye damage may be decreased by taking vitamin D supplements.

3. limiting exposure to smoking

Smoking has been shown to raise the risk of developing eye issues by seven to eight times and is a significant factor in disease severity6. Additionally, it makes your responses to therapy worse.

The single best thing you can do to lessen Graves' ophthalmopathy symptoms is to stop smoking if you do.

The cornea, which is the transparent front part of your eye, as well as the tear film are both harmed by secondhand smoke, which can also interfere with natural lubrication.

Further eye irritation can be avoided by giving up smoking and limiting exposure to secondhand smoke.

4. Methods of eye relief from the outside

You can find relief from mild cases of Graves' ophthalmopathy by using straightforward, non-invasive treatments.

External therapies' primary objectives are to lessen dry eyes and stop corneal damage. Typical treatments include:.

5. Eye drops that lubricate

These can aid in healthy blinking and lubricate dry, scratchy eyes. Drops without preservatives offer a more all-natural treatment and lower the chance of irritation.

- compress that is chilly.
- The pain and swelling around the eyes can be reduced with a cold compress.
- taped-close eyes for sleep.

When eyelid swelling prevents eyes from closing, taping the eyes before bed can help prevent the dryness that comes from having the inner eye exposed to air for a long time. Find out from your doctor how to properly tape your eyes.

In the evening, elevate your head.

At night, higher pillows or more pillows are helpful. The ability to drain fluid from the face and lessen swelling can both benefit from sleeping with the head elevated.

Sunglasses

Eyes that have become sensitive to light are shielded by sunglasses. Wraparound styles will also guard against airflow across the eye's surface irritation.

The Fresnel prism glasses

To assist wearers in controlling double vision, these plastic prisms stick to the front of the glasses. However, these only improve vision when you are wearing glasses.

Vision treatment

Under the supervision of a qualified medical professional, this procedure is carried out. Retraining the brain-to-eye pathways and enhancing visual abilities are accomplished through exercises.

Thyroid hyperfunction and Graves' disease

Thyroid hormone issues arise when the thyroid gland produces either an excessive amount or insufficient amounts of thyroid hormone.

Hyperthyroidism is brought on by the thyroid's overactive release of thyroid hormone into the bloodstream. The body consumes energy more quickly than it should, and cell metabolism and other chemical processes quicken.

Hypothyroidism results from the thyroid producing too little thyroid hormone when it is underactive. The body's energy consumption slows down along with the cells' chemical activity, or metabolism.

What Are the Symptoms and Signs of Hyperthyroidism?

Hyperthyroidism, or elevated levels of thyroid hormones, can lead to:

- nervousness
- irritability.
- a greater sweating.
- wide eyes.
- issues with sleep
- a rapid heart rate
- irregular girls' periods

- loss of weight

- A goiter, a swelling in the neck caused by the thyroid gland, can occasionally develop

Hyperthyroidism can be successfully treated with medications and other methods. It's crucial to work with an endocrinologist or another medical professional with experience in treating thyroid issues.

Why Does Hyperthyroidism Occur?

These are the top three causes of hyperthyroidism.

Graves disease: The most frequent reason for hyperthyroidism in kids is this. The thyroid gland becomes overactive as a result of the body producing antibodies. Antibodies typically aid the body's defense against infection, but in some cases, they prevent the body from properly controlling the thyroid gland (much like a car without brakes). Thyroid hormone levels can thus rise to extremely high levels in the blood. The reason the body begins producing these antibodies is unknown to medical professionals. For the rest of a person's life, Graves' disease can have an impact on their health. To control it, it's crucial to receive medical care.

Thyroiditis: An inflammation of the thyroid gland. The thyroid gland as a result secretes an excessive amount of thyroid hormone into the blood. There are numerous factors that can lead to thyroiditis, including trauma to the thyroid gland, infections, and autoimmune conditions like Hashimoto's thyroiditis. Thyroiditis-related hyperthyroidism typically lasts for a few months before clearing up on its own. Although the thyroid usually recovers, sometimes it suffers damage and cannot function normally once more. Hypothyroidism (underactive thyroid) is brought on by this.

growths on the thyroid gland called thyroid nodules. These can occasionally produce a lot of thyroid hormones, which can result in hyperthyroidism symptoms. Usually large (an inch or larger in size), overactive thyroid nodules can be felt in the neck. Surgery is used to treat the majority of benign overactive thyroid nodules.

What Indicates a Graves' Disease Diagnosis?

Children and adolescents who have Graves' disease might observe that:

- More so than usual, they are exhausted.
- They have a difficult time falling asleep.
- They slim down.
- Their heart is pumping quickly.
- They have tremors in their hands.
- They struggle a lot to concentrate

Sometimes Graves' disease-affected girls notice that their menstrual cycles are shorter or less regular. Many people become aware of their enlarge thyroid glands over time.

Itching, burning, redness, and occasionally difficulty seeing normally are symptoms of Graves' disease that some individuals experience in their eyes. Sometimes they experience eye pressure, eye bulge, or double vision. Inflammation and swelling behind the eyes are brought on by the same antibodies that cause the thyroid to become overactive. It is known as Graves' eye disease when this occurs.

How is Graves' disease identified?

A doctor will review the patient's symptoms and conduct an examination to determine whether Graves' disease is present.

Furthermore, since many people can experience some of the symptoms of hyperthyroidism for unrelated conditions, it is crucial to perform lab tests. Sometimes additional tests, such as an ultrasound or thyroid scan, are required because the results of the blood tests alone cannot always be relied upon to make a diagnosis.

How Is Graves' Disease Managed?

Typically, anti-thyroid medications are used by doctors to treat Graves' disease.

These drugs reduce the thyroid gland's ability to release thyroid hormones. They usually bring hormone levels down to normal within a couple of months.

For a very long time, sometimes for the rest of their lives, many people with Graves disease must take anti-thyroid medications to control the condition.

Some might need other treatment if anti-thyroid medicines don't help or cause side effects, or if the disease is very hard to control. In these cases, two permanent treatment options can be used: radioactive iodine treatment and surgery.

The most popular long-term remedy for Graves' disease is radioactive iodine (RAI)

Surgery to remove most of the thyroid gland is called a thyroidectomy. It's done in a hospital under general anesthesia, so the person is asleep and feels nothing. A small incision (cut) in the lower central part of the neck usually leaves a thin scar. It's common to have some pain for a few days after the surgery, but most people feel much better within a few days.

After treatment for hyperthyroidism, hormone production often slows down to hypothyroid (underactive) levels. So the person needs to take a thyroid hormone replacement tablet each day. This treatment is a lot easier to manage than taking pills to control the hyperthyroidism — fewer blood tests, doctor visits, and medicine changes are needed.

As the body adjusts to the hormone replacement tablets, a doctor may increase or reduce the dosage until the levels of thyroid hormone are normal. When the doctor finds the proper dosage, people usually feel well and free of symptoms. The doctor will continue to check hormone levels to make sure the dosage is right, especially for growing teens whose levels might change over just a few months.

What Else Should I Know?
We don't know why people develop Graves' disease. But with good medical

help, kids and teens can be healthy and do all the things other kids and teens can do.

Graves' eye disease can develop at any time in someone who has Graves' disease. Smoke can make this eye disease much worse, so it's very important to not smoke and to avoid secondhand smoke.

Women with Graves' disease need to be very careful to keep their hormone levels in balance. Uncontrolled thyroid hormone levels in a pregnant woman can lead to problems during pregnancy and harm her baby.

What are the symptoms of Graves' disease and how is it diagnosed?
The thyroid plays a critical role in metabolism. When, as in Graves' disease, it makes too much thyroid hormone, the

body's metabolism is greatly accelerated. This results in symptoms of hyperthyroidism, which can begin mildly with anxiety, distracted attention, nervousness, irritability, heat intolerance, and difficulty sleeping. Gradually, a patient can begin to become fatigued, experiencing a rapid or irregular heartbeat, shaking, increased perspiration, changes in libido, weight loss despite normal food intake, brittle hair, frequent bowel movements, and in women, light menstrual periods. In some cases, the tissue and muscles behind the eyes swells, making them bulge. The skin near the ankles may also develop a thick red rash.

If a thyroid anomaly is suspected, blood tests are usually performed to determine levels of thyroid-stimulating hormone

(TSH) and thyroxine, one of the circulating thyroid hormones. TSH, produced by the pituitary gland, is the hormone that normally stimulates the thyroid. In Graves' disease, abnormal antibodies are present in the blood, which are detectable and mimic the actions of TSH, causing elevated thyroxine even while natural TSH levels remain low.

A radioactive thyroid uptake exam can also be done to assess thyroid function. The body needs iodine to make thyroid hormone; and by ingesting a small amount of radiolabeled iodine, then later measuring how much of it is taken into the thyroid, a doctor can see how well the gland is producing. High iodine uptake indicates that the thyroid is making too much hormone, as is the case in Graves' disease.

What are the causes?

In Graves' disease, the immune system mistakenly targets the thyroid gland, making a faulty antibody (TRAb) that stimulates the thyroid to make excessive amounts of hormone. The thyroid is normally tightly regulated by areas of the brain – the pituitary gland and hypothalamus – that tell it to appropriately turn on and off. This antibody interrupts the normal feedback mechanism that regulates production of adequate amounts of thyroid hormone, causing levels to be abnormally high. We still don't know what factors may precipitate the immune system to attack the thyroid gland. There does seem to be a genetic component, as Graves' is found more commonly in certain families and in twins. Other risks, such as gender – it occurs more in women – and age (it usually affects people over the age of 20) also play a role. Recent illness or infections, as well as stress, are additionally linked with developing Graves' disease.

What is the conventional treatment?
An overactive thyroid is initially treated with radioactive iodine taken orally (as a capsule or drink). The radiation helps to shrink the gland and permanently reduce its hormone output within three to six months. (Radioactive iodine rarely has side effects, and all the radioactivity is eliminated in the urine within two to three

days.) . Sometimes anti-thyroid drugs such as propylthiouracil or methimazole (Tapazole) may be given initially to reduce hormone levels; in about a third of cases, taking these medications for a year or more can produce a long-term remission. Still, relapse is common, prompting patients to seek out radioactive iodine treatment. Dr. Weil suggests these proven therapies be considered before having all or part of the thyroid gland surgically removed. Risks of this surgery can include potential damage to the vocal cords and the parathyroid glands, tiny glands located adjacent to the thyroid that control calcium absorption. Following thyroid surgery or treatment with radioactive iodine, people frequently develop low levels of thyroid hormone, becoming hypothyroid in the process and needing long-term thyroid hormone replacement. Graves' disease is a more serious condition than an underactive thyroid since the rapid heartbeat it can cause can progress to other serious heart problems if not adequately treated.

Beta blockers, including propranolol (Inderal), atenolol (Tenormin), and metoprolol (Lopressor) can often relieve the rapid heart rate, nervousness and tremors that come from an overactive thyroid. These medications aren't a cure for Graves' because the body will still overproduce thyroid hormone, but they can block some of its action. Beta blockers are often used with other forms of treatment until or unless thyroid function stops or becomes too low.

Dietary changes: Decrease protein intake toward 10 percent of daily calories; replace animal protein as much as possible with plant protein, see the anti-inflammatory food pyramid.

Eliminate milk and milk products, substituting other calcium sources.

Eat more fruits and vegetables regularly; make sure they are organically grown.

Eliminate polyunsaturated vegetable oils, margarine, vegetable shortening, all partially hydrogentated oils, and all foods (such as deep-fried foods) that might contain trans-fatty acids. Use extra-virgin olive oil as your main fat.

Mind/Body: Mind-body measures like guided imagery and hypnosis are worth practicing to help reduce stress and normalize immune function, but it's not clear if such methods will lessen symptoms. Dr. Gary Conrad, an integrative medicine colleague, has written an excellent article published in the November/December, 2007, issue of Explore magazine entitled: Spontaneous Remission of Graves' **Disease:** A Spiritual Odyssey. Dr. Conrad recommends the use of a multisystem, integrative approach that encompasses "all healing modalities" most appropriate to address an individual's needs. One key component to his healing was learning how to optimize the mind-body connection to achieve states of deep relaxation – what Dr. Conrad calls the "opposite of Graves' Disease" – along with accessing the inner healing wisdom of the body to give insight about further treatment options. Dr.

Conrad's article makes two key points about autoimmune conditions like Graves' disease. First, they can go into spontaneous remission over time – a focus of treatment should be trying to get the condition to "burn itself out. " Secondly, stress is often a key precipitator in aggravating these conditions, and working to decrease or better manage stress can often balance immune system function and facilitate healing.

What Is Graves' Disease?

Graves' disease is an autoimmune condition that causes your thyroid to become hyperactive -- work harder than it needs to. It is one of the most common thyroid problems and the leading cause of hyperthyroidism, a condition in which the thyroid gland produces too many hormones. It was named after the man who first described it in the early 19th century, Sir Robert Graves.

The thyroid gland is a small butterfly-shaped gland that sits in the front of your neck and releases hormones that help regulate your metabolism. When you have Graves' disease, your immune system attacks your thyroid, causing it to overproduce those hormones, which causes a number of problems in different parts of your body. It usually affects people between the ages of 30 and 50 and is more common in women.

Once the disorder has been correctly diagnosed, it is quite easy to treat. In some cases, Graves' disease goes into remission or disappears completely after several months or years. Left untreated, however, it can lead to serious complications -- even death.

Causes of Graves' Disease

Graves' disease. Graves' disease is an autoimmune disease in which your thyroid works harder than it needs to (hyperthyroidism). Some patients develop thyroid eye disease in which their eye muscles and tissues swell, causing the eyes to protrude from their sockets (exophthalmos).

Normally, the thyroid gets its production orders through another chemical called thyroid-stimulating hormone (TSH), released by the pituitary gland in the brain. But in Graves' disease, a malfunction in the body's immune system releases abnormal antibodies that act like TSH. Spurred by these false signals to produce, the thyroid's hormone factories work overtime and overproduce.

Exactly why the immune system begins to produce these troublesome antibodies isn't clear. Heredity and other characteristics seem to play a role. Studies show, for example, that if one identical twin contracts Graves' disease, there is a 20 percent likelihood that the other twin will get it too. Also, women are more likely than men to develop the disease. And smokers who develop Graves' disease are more prone to eye problems than nonsmokers with the disease. No single gene causes Graves' disease. It is thought to be triggered by both genetics and environmental factors.

Symptoms of Graves' Disease

The most common symptoms of Graves' are symptoms of hyperthyroidism, which include:

- Nervousness, anxiety or irritability.
- Tired or weak muscles.
- Shaking in your hands.
- Frequent bowel movements or diarrhea.
- Difficulty sleeping.
- Greater sensitivity to heat or increase sweating.
- Unintentional weight loss.
- An enlarged thyroid (also called a goiter).

RAI damages the thyroid gland so that it can't make too much thyroid hormone.

This doesn't harm other parts of the body.

The RAI treatment is taken in capsules or mixed with a glass of water.

The thyroid gland quickly absorbs the RAI from the bloodstream and, within a few months, the gland shrinks and symptoms slowly disappear.

- an erratic or quick heartbeat.
- changes to a woman's menstrual cycle.
- male impotence.
- low libido or loss of sex drive.
- Graves' disease complications.

Problems with the eyes

Thyroid eye disease, which causes swollen eye muscles and tissues, affects a small percentage of all Graves' disease patients. Even though it's uncommon, this can lead to exophthalmos, a condition in which your eyes protrude from their sockets, and is regarded as a sign of Graves' disease. However, whether you have this complication has nothing to do with how severe your Graves' disease is. It is actually unclear whether these eye complications are caused by Graves' disease specifically or by a completely unrelated but closely related disorder. Your eyes may hurt, feel dry, and irritated if you have thyroid eye disease. Due in part to the eyelids' inability to adequately shield protruding eyeballs, they are more prone to excessive tearing and redness.

Rarely, severe exophthalmos can cause swollen eye muscles to put a great deal of pressure on the optic nerve, potentially causing partial blindness. Double vision can occur when eye muscles that have been overly stressed by prolonged inflammation are unable to control movement.

Complications with the skin

Pretibial myxedema, also referred to as Graves' dermopathy, can occur in some Graves' disease sufferers. The skin on the shins has thickened in a lumpy, reddish pattern. Typically, there is no pain and there is no danger. Similar to exophthalmos, this condition doesn't necessarily start when Graves' disease does and has nothing to do with how severe your disease is.

Identification of Graves' disease

Your doctor will likely ask you if you have a family history of the condition and order one or more of the following tests if you exhibit symptoms or signs of Graves' disease complications.

Thyroid stimulating hormone (TSH) and other thyroid hormone levels can be checked through a blood test. Your TSH levels are typically suppressed and your other hormone levels are elevated if you have Graves' disease.

the antibodies that cause Graves' disease will be tested in the lab. If you don't have them, your hyperthyroidism is likely brought on by something else.

A radioactive iodine uptake test measures how much radioactive iodine is absorbed into your thyroid from your bloodstream using small doses of radioactive iodine. If you consume a lot of the radioactive iodine, your body is working harder than it needs to because it normally uses iodine to make thyroid hormones.

a thyroid scan to track the movement of radioactive iodine inside your thyroid gland. Since other causes of hypothyroidism only affect some portions of the gland, if it affects your entire thyroid, that suggests you have Graves' disease.

Treatment for Graves' disease

The treatment for Graves' disease has two objectives. One is to prevent your thyroid from producing too much thyroid hormone. The second is to prevent issues with your body from developing as a result of the elevated levels of thyroid hormone. To accomplish one or both of these objectives, there are various treatment options.

Treatment with radioactive iodine

In order to receive this treatment, you must consume a different type of radioactive iodine than that which is used in the Graves' disease test. A portion of the thyroid cells that are overproducing thyroid hormones are killed by the radiation after the iodine enters the thyroid. This treatment may temporarily exacerbate any Graves' disease-related eye issues you may have, and it will probably result in lower-than-normal thyroid hormone production. Your low thyroid can be treated if that occurs. Radiation is used in this treatment, so it is not recommended for use on women who are pregnant or nursing.

Medications

Anti-thyroid drugs reduce thyroid hormone production from your thyroid. Although they can be used for a long time and occasionally even after you have stopped treatment, they are not permanent treatments. For women who can't be exposed to radiation because they are pregnant or nursing, they are typically the treatment of choice. Additionally, radioactive iodine therapy is occasionally combined with them.

Beta blockers are typically used to lower blood pressure, but they can also help quickly alleviate some hyperthyroidism symptoms like anxiety, trembling, and fast heartbeat.

Surgery is a less common Graves' disease treatment, but it might be a good option if you have a goiter or you can't take anti-thyroid medications because you're pregnant. Your thyroid gland may be partially or completely removed during surgery. You might need to take daily thyroid medication for the rest of your life after surgery.

Graves' disease generally has no long-term detrimental health effects if you receive prompt and appropriate medical care, despite the fact that the symptoms can be uncomfortable.

Graves disease

The overproduction of thyroid hormones (hyperthyroidism) is a symptom of Graves' disease, an immune system disorder. Graves' disease is a common cause of hyperthyroidism, though a variety of illnesses can also result in it.

The signs and symptoms of Graves' disease can vary widely because thyroid hormones have an impact on numerous bodily systems. Although anyone can develop Graves' disease, it is more prevalent in women and in people under the age of 40.

The body's production of thyroid hormones is to be decreased, and the severity of symptoms is to be decreased.

Graves' disease is frequently accompanied by the following signs and symptoms:

- Angry and anxious.
- a slight shuddering of the fingers or hands.
- Heat sensitivity, an increase in perspiration, or warm, damp skin.
- Despite regular eating habits, weight loss.
- Goiter, an enlargement of the thyroid gland.
- alterations to menstrual cycles.

- a diminished libido or erectile dysfunction.
- frequent bathroom visits.
- Eyes that are swollen (Graves' ophthalmopathy).
- Fatigue.

Graves' dermopathy is characterized by thick, red skin that typically affects the shins or tops of the feet.

- palpitations, a rapid or erratic heartbeat.
- disturbance in sleep.
- ophthalmopathy caused by Graves.

INCIDENCES OF GRAVES' DISEASE THAT AFFECT THE EYES

Obstructive Graves' disease

The Graves ophthalmopathy is manifested in about 30% of Graves' disease patients. Muscles and other tissues around your eyes are impacted by inflammation and other immune system events in Graves' ophthalmopathy. Among the warning signs and symptoms are:

- eyes that are swollen.
- I feel something scratchy in my eyes.
- The eyes may feel tight or painful.
- eyelids that are droopy or retracted.
- eyes that are swollen or red.
- light responsiveness.

- Multiple vision.

- vision impairment.

- Dermopathy associated with Graves.

- Dermopathy due to Graves.

Dermopathy associated with Graves

The reddening and thickening of the skin, known as Graves' dermopathy, is an uncommon Graves' disease symptom that most frequently affects the tops of your feet or shins.

When to visit the doctor

The Graves' disease-related signs and symptoms can be brought on by a variety of medical conditions. For a prompt and precise diagnosis if you suspect you may be suffering from Graves' disease, consult your doctor.

Causes

A breakdown in the immune system, which the body uses to fight disease, is the root cause of Graves' disease. Why this occurs is a mystery.

Antibodies produced by the immune system are typically intended to attack a particular virus, bacterium, or other foreign substance. For unknown reasons, the immune system creates an antibody against a portion of the cells in the thyroid gland, a neck-based gland that produces hormones, in Graves' disease.

Normally, a hormone produced by the pituitary gland, a small gland at the base of the brain, controls how the thyroid works. Thyrotropin receptor antibody (TRAb), an antibody linked to Graves' disease, functions similarly to the regulatory pituitary hormone. This means that TRAb interferes with the thyroid's natural regulation, leading to an excessive production of thyroid hormones (hyperthyroidism).

Origin of Graves' ophthalmopathy

The cause of Graves' ophthalmopathy, which results from a buildup of particular carbohydrates in the muscles and tissues behind the eyes, is unknown. It seems that the same antibody that can lead to thyroid dysfunction may also have an "attraction" to tissues around the eyes.

When hyperthyroidism first manifests, or a few months later, Graves' ophthalmopathy frequently follows. However, ophthalmopathy symptoms and signs may manifest years before or after the onset of hyperthyroidism. If there is no hyperthyroidism, Graves' ophthalmopathy can still happen.

Risk elements

Although Graves' disease can affect anyone, a number of things can make it more likely to occur, including:

1. History of the family

Given that a family history of Graves' disease is a known risk factor, the disorder is probably caused by one or more genes.

2. Sex

Compared to men, women have a significantly higher risk of developing Graves' disease.

3. Age

People under the age of 40 typically develop Graves' disease.

Additional autoimmune conditions.
A higher risk exists in those who have other immune system diseases like type 1 diabetes or rheumatoid arthritis.

psychological or physical strain. In those with genes that increase their risk of developing Graves' disease, stressful life events or illness may be the catalyst for the disease's onset.

1. Pregnancy

In particular among women who have genes that increase their risk, pregnancy or recent childbirth may raise the risk of the disorder.

2. Smoking

The risk of Graves' disease is increased by cigarette smoking, which can have an adverse impact on the immune system. Smokers with Graves' disease are more likely to develop Gravesophthalmopathy.

Complications

Graves' disease side effects can consist of:

1. Pregnancy-related problems

Miscarriage, premature birth, fetal thyroid dysfunction, poor fetal growth, maternal heart failure, and preeclampsia are all potential side effects of Graves' disease during pregnancy. A maternal condition called preeclampsia causes high blood pressure along with other serious symptoms.

2. heart conditions

Graves' disease can cause heart rhythm problems, modifications to the way the heart muscles look and work, and heart failure, which is when the heart is unable to pump enough blood to the body.

3. Storming of the thyroid

Thyroid storm, also referred to as accelerated hyperthyroidism or thyrotoxic crisis, is a rare but serious side effect of Graves' disease. When severe hyperthyroidism is untreated or improperly treated, the likelihood increases.

Numerous effects, such as fever, sweating, vomiting, diarrhea, delirium, extreme weakness, seizures, irregular heartbeat, yellow skin and eyes (jaundice), severely low blood pressure, and coma, can result from the sudden and drastic increase in thyroid hormones. Emergency care must be given right away for thyroid storm.

broken bones. Osteoporosis, another side effect of untreated hyperthyroidism, can cause fragile, brittle bones. The calcium and other minerals that make up your bones play a role in how strong they are. The ability of your body to incorporate calcium into your bones is hampered by an excess of thyroid hormone.

Causes of Graves disease

It seems unclear what specifically causes Grave's disease. According to theory, Graves' disease is an autoimmune condition that causes hyperthyroidism or excessive thyroid activity.

What exactly does the thyroid gland do?

The thyroid is a tiny, butterfly-shaped gland that produces the hormones triiodothyronine (T3) and thyroxine (T4) and is located in front of the voice box on the neck. These hormones aid in controlling the body's important processes like metabolism, brain development, heart rate, energy levels, and calorie burning.

Overall, the thyroid hormones maintain a delicate balance in controlling mood, weight, and mental and physical energy levels.

The condition is known as hyperthyroidism when there is an excess of these hormones, and as hypothyroidism when there is a deficiency of these hormones.

What does autoimmune disease mean?

When a person has an autoimmune condition, their immune system's defenses against foreign microbes or other organisms turn against their own tissues. These cells produce antibodies that are directed against the target tissues, which can cause those tissues to deteriorate or become ill.

Graves' disease's root causes

In Graves' disease, the body begins to produce antibodies that cause the thyroid gland to produce more hormone than usual. The main factor causing hyperthyroidism is Graves' disease.

Thyroid-stimulating immunoglobulins (TSIs), which are produced by the B and T lymphocytes at this point, are antibodies directed against the thyroid gland. The thyroid contains 4 distinct proteins that these antibodies are designed to attack. Among them are:

- Thyroglobulin.
- thyroxine peroxidase

- Sodium-iodide synporter

Receptor for thyroid stimulating hormone (TSH)

Thyroid stimulating hormone (TSH) causes the thyroid to produce T3 and T4 hormones under normal circumstances by acting on tiny receptors over the thyroid gland. the initial antibody that results in.

The condition that targets the TSH receptor is Graves disease

The antibodies act like thyroid-stimulating hormone (TSH) and bind to the thyroid cell's TSH receptor, which causes the thyroid gland to enlarge and swell, resulting in a goiter. Additionally, the thyroid follicles are stimulated by these antibodies to produce more thyroid hormone. The symptoms of hyperthyroidism result from this.

The three other antibodies may be tested to track the course of the disease even though they play a less significant part in the pathophysiology of Graves' disease. A small percentage of people with TSI and anti-thyroid peroxidase antibodies may also develop hypothyroidism over time— about 5%. This indicates that their thyroid gland secretes less hormone than is required. Hypothyroidism may also result when patients' antibodies block rather than stimulate the TSH receptors.

Who is affected by Graves' disease?

Autoimmune diseases are more common in women. When compared to men, women can have Graves up to eight times more frequently. A person is also more likely to develop Graves' disease if they have another autoimmune disorder, such as pernicious anemia, vitiligo, rheumatoid arthritis, or insulin-dependent diabetes, or if a family member has one of these conditions.

Between the ages of 20 and 40, the disease most frequently affects people. Graves' disease, however, can also affect men and people of other ages.

Graves' disease and genes

The risk of developing Graves' disease may also be influenced by genes. The condition appears to run in some families as some have multiple cases.

It has been hypothesized that genes encoding for CD40, CTLA-4, thyroglobulin, TSH receptor, and PTPN22 may pass the condition from parents to children. It has been discovered which specific gene loci. These may vary between various racial and ethnic groups.

Environmental elements and the disease of Graves.
It has also been discovered that some bacteria, including Gram-negative organisms like Yersinia enterocolitica, Escherichia coli, and others, have TSH binding sites. In addition, thyroid issues could result from these.

Included in the list of environmental causes of thyroid conditions like Graves' disease is:

- smoking.

- stress.

- pollution.

- pregnancy.

- therapy with iodine.

- intake of selenium.

- thyroid gland damage or thyroid surgery.

- the injection of specific drugs like ethanol, interferon beta-1b, interleukin-4 therapy, etc.

Why Does Graves' Disease Occur?

In autoimmune disorders like Graves' disease, the body makes antibodies that it uses to fight against itself.

Hyperthyroidism, or an overproduction of thyroid hormones, may result from this.

Autoimmunity is the primary cause of Graves' disease. Numerous biological and environmental factors have been shown to activate specific genes linked to autoimmune disease, though the precise cause is unknown. The activation of these genes, according to medical professionals, raises the risk of developing Graves' disease.

Any genetic factor, even some biological factors, cannot be avoided or altered. But being aware of the mutable environmental factors causing Graves' disease may inspire you to adopt a more wholesome way of life.

So what is the cause of Graves' disease?

When antibodies prompt the immune system to attack the body's healthy cells, autoimmune disease results.

Some significant immune system elements found in the blood that may contribute to Graves' disease are described using the terms below:

Toxins, bacteria, and viruses are just a few examples of the foreign substances that antibodies attach to and remove. They accomplish this by attaching to a particular antigen and destroying it.

Foreign substances known as antigens attach to antibodies or T cell receptors to be eliminated and destroyed. They are the ones who start immune reactions.

Specific antibodies are produced by B cells, which are specialized cells.

Directly destroying foreign virus- or bacteria-infected cells are cytotoxic T cells.

Our B cells are stimulated by helper T cells to produce antibodies

Autoimmune process

The autoimmune process that results in Graves' disease develops as follows:.

1. The normal mechanism the body employs to prevent autoimmune reactions has a flaw for some reason (likely genetic).
2. The thyroid gland contains an antigen, which causes the T cells to

react overly strongly to it, allowing them to grow.

3. The thyroid gland cells contain antigens that the B cells are stimulated to produce antibodies (TRAb) against because they mistakenly perceive these antigens as foreign invaders.

4. These antibodies bind to thyroid-stimulating hormone (TSH) receptors found on thyroid cell surfaces. They cause the receptor to be activated, producing a response similar to what TSH would have done had the thyroid been operating normally.

5. This reaction may lead to:

- the excessive secretion of thyroid hormones (T3 and T4) into the bloodstream and their production.

- thyroid gland enlargement (goiter).
- progression to the condition known as "Graves' ophthalmopathy.
- Risk components.

In spite of the fact that our immune system has evolved to guard against autoimmune reactions, genetic and environmental factors can still override this.

Although the precise cause of antibodies attacking our healthy cells is unknown, many different factors are thought to be possible.

It is not the cause of Graves' disease to have these risk factors. You still do not necessarily have Graves' disease if you have one or more risk factors. However, having specific genes increases your risk of getting Graves' disease, especially if you're also exposed to certain environmental factors.

DNA and family history

A third1 or more of people with Graves' disease have relatives who also have the condition or another autoimmune thyroid disorder called "Hashimoto's disease.". ' .

According to a study of twins, genetic factors may account for about 80% of a person's1 risk of Graves' disease. Genetically predisposed individuals may experience immune defects that result in the overproduction of thyroid hormones and antibodies, which in turn causes the thyroid gland to enlarge.

Aspects of the environment

Environmental factors raise the risk of getting Graves' disease, and experts estimate that they account for 20% of cases.

Immune responses in the genes linked to Graves' disease (listed above) are probably triggered by environmental factors.

Among the crucial environmental elements are:

1. Trauma or stress on a psychological level

Studies have suggested a link between Graves' disease and prior trauma2.

However, it is unknown what causes this to happen.

In people with Graves' disease, stress is also thought to be a factor in determining the severity[3] of the hyperthyroidism symptoms. The effectiveness of the treatment may also be hampered by stress.

Thyroid autoantibodies, however, are not associated with stress per se. For those who are genetically predisposed to the condition, stress is more likely to set off the hyperthyroidism that leads to Graves' disease.

2. Smoking cigarettes

Smoking increases the likelihood of getting Graves' disease by twofold[4] and is associated with worsening symptoms.

Graves' ophthalmopathy risk is also increased by threefold.

People who have a genetic predisposition to Graves' disease are more likely to exhibit this relationship.

Smoking, according to experts, may reduce the thyroid gland's resistance to infection.

3. Infections

Diseases like H. Graves' disease may be exacerbated by pylori, a bacterial infection of the mucous membrane lining the stomach.

Considered to be the H.

Pylori antigens may contribute to the onset of autoimmune thyroid disease.

The onset of Graves' disease is also linked to Yersinia enterocoliticainfection.

4. Iodine exposure

Iodine is a crucial mineral that aids in the production of thyroid hormones by the thyroid gland. A risk factor for Graves' disease, however, is excessive iodine exposure, which can cause hyperthyroidism.

Studies suggest that too much iodine may worsen thyroid autoimmunity.

Additionally, excessive iodine exposure may lessen the efficiency of antithyroid medications used to treat Graves' disease.

Pregnancy and the time after childbirth

There is a 1–5% chance that women with Graves' disease now or in the past will pass the condition to their unborn child and cause fetal hyperthyroidism.

Women who stopped treatment for hyperthyroidism during their pregnancy are more likely to develop postpartum Graves disease, which can appear three to nine months after giving birth.

Drug treatment

antiretroviral therapy that is extremely active (HAART).

HIV treatment known as HAART. It has been demonstrated that 8 to 12 months after beginning this medication, Graves' disease can appear.

1. IL-1 alpha cytokine

This therapy is crucial in minimizing joint damage and inflammation in Graves' disease.

2. IL-2 and IFN alfa cytokines

Chemotherapy uses the anti-inflammatory agents interleukin-2 (IL-2) and interferon alpha (IFN-alpha). They can worsen autoimmune thyroid disorders4 or even cause them by directly affecting the thyroid.

3. The Campath

A unique class of antibody called campath is used to treat MS.

One-third of MS patients who were recovering from T-cell depletion in a study experienced the onset of Graves' disease within six months.

Neck area exposure to radiation

Graves' disease and Gravesophthalmopathy are more likely to develop after exposure to radiation in the neck region, such as during treatment for Hodgkin's disease.

Additional Biological Variables

Gender

Various autoimmune diseases, including Graves' disease, are more common in women. The female sex hormone estrogen is thought by experts to be connected to this correlation.

an immune system that is currently ineffective, e.g. arthritis, and diabetes.

An individual's risk of getting Graves' disease can rise if they also have other autoimmune diseases. Among them are type 1 diabetes and rheumatoid arthritis.

Why does Graves' disease relapse?

Even though Graves' disease is treatable, relapse is always a possibility. 50% of patients6 relapse even after successfully using antithyroid medications as treatment.

Similar to the original disease's causes, Graves' disease relapses have similar causes. But a few things could make the risk of relapse even higher.

Even though each individual factor has only a small impact, a review of studies revealed some factors that could predict relapse before Graves' disease treatment has even started. These consist of:

- the act of smoking.
- young male status.

- having a large thyroid or goiter.

- when first diagnosed with severe hyperthyroidism.

- Thyroid autoantibodies at high and prolonged levels after treatment.

- the occurrence of orbitopathy, which causes the eyes to bulge as a result of swelling behind the eyes.

Ophthalmopathyand dermopathy associated with Graves.

Graves' disease is closely related to Graves' dermopathy and Graves' ophthalmopathy.

Around 30% of people with Graves' disease experience Graves' ophthalmopathy. But Graves' dermopathy is much less frequent.

Both of these illnesses are autoimmune responses, just like Graves' disease.

Ocular Graves disease

TSH receptors can also be found in the muscles and connective tissue around the eyes, in addition to the thyroid. Inflammation, swelling, scarring, and an outward bulging of the eye result from a specific antibody (thyroid-stimulating immunoglobulin) binding to a TSH receptor on the surface of cells behind the eye.

Dermopathydue to Graves.

Similar to Graves' ophthalmopathy, doctors think that TSHR receptors in the connective tissue beneath the skin function as an antigen and trigger an immune response. On the shins and the tops of the feet in particular, this results in red, swollen, and thickened skin.

GRAVES' ILLNESS

Diagnosis

Your doctor may perform a physical examination and look for Graves' disease symptoms to make the diagnosis. He or she might also talk about your health and family background.

Aside from these, your doctor might also recommend:

testing with blood. Your doctor can determine your thyroid hormone levels and thyroid-stimulating hormone (TSH) levels using blood tests. TSH is a hormone produced by the pituitary gland that normally stimulates the thyroid gland. TSH levels are frequently below normal and thyroid hormone levels are elevated in people with Graves' disease.

The levels of the antibody known to cause Graves' disease may be determined by a different lab test that your doctor may order for you. Although results that don't show antibodies may point to another cause of hyperthyroidism, the disease is typically not necessary to diagnose.

Iodine uptake from radiation

The production of thyroid hormones by your body requires iodine.

Your doctor can ascertain the rate at which your thyroid gland absorbs iodine by administering you a small quantity of radioactive iodine, and then measuring the amount of it in your thyroid gland with a specialized scanning camera. Determine whether Graves' disease or another condition is the cause of the hyperthyroidism by measuring the amount

137

of radioactive iodine the thyroid gland absorbs. For a visual representation of the uptake pattern, this test may be combined with a radioactive iodine scan.

Ultrasound

To create images of the structures inside the body, ultrasound uses high-frequency sound waves. It can demonstrate whether the thyroid gland is enlarged. It is most helpful for those who can't undergo radioactive iodine uptake, like pregnant women.

image-based tests. Your doctor may recommend specialized imaging tests, such as a CT scan or MRI, if it is unclear whether Graves' disease has been diagnosed based solely on a clinical evaluation.

138

Treatment

Stopping the production of thyroid hormones and blocking their impact on the body are the main goals of treatment for Graves' disease. Some therapies consist of:

Radiation therapy with iodine

You take radioactive iodine (radioiodine) orally during this therapy. The thyroid absorbs radioiodine into the thyroid cells because it needs iodine to produce hormones, and the radiation gradually kills the overactive thyroid cells. As a result, your thyroid gland shrinks and your symptoms gradually get better over several weeks to months.

You run a greater risk of developing new or worsening Graves' ophthalmopathy symptoms if you receive radioiodine therapy. If you already have moderate to severe eye problems, the therapy might not be advised even though this side effect is typically mild and transient.

Tenderness in the neck and a brief rise in thyroid hormones are possible additional side effects. Women who are pregnant or nursing are not treated with radioiodine therapy.

You'll probably need treatment later to give your body the normal amount of thyroid hormones because this treatment lowers thyroid activity.

Medicines that block the thyroid
Anti-thyroid drugs prevent the thyroid from using iodine to make hormones. These prescription drugs include

methimazole (Tapazole) and propylthiouracil.

When prescribing medication, methimazole is typically the first option because propylthiouracil has a higher prevalence of liver disease risk. However, because methimazole carries a small risk of birth defects, propylthiouracil is the preferred anti-thyroid medication during the first trimester of pregnancy. Typically, after the first trimester, pregnant women resume taking methimazole.

A relapse of hyperthyroidism may happen down the road if these two medications are used in isolation without other therapies. Better long-term effects might be attained by using either medication for more than a year. As an additional form of treatment, anti-thyroid medications may be used prior to or following radioiodine therapy.

Rash, joint pain, liver failure, or a reduction in white blood cells that fight infection are just a few of the side effects that both medications can cause.

Beta adsorbents
The effects of hormones on the body are blocked by these medications, but they do not prevent the production of thyroid hormones. Insomnia, tremors, anxiety, irritability, heat intolerance, sweating, diarrhea, and muscle weakness may all be fairly quickly relievedby them.

Among the beta blockers are:

- Inderal, InnoPran XL are brands of propranolol.
- Tenormin, or atenolol.
- Metoprolol (brand names: Lopressor and Toprol-XL).
- Naddolol (Corgard).

Since beta blockers have the potential to precipitate an asthma attack, they are not frequently prescribed to asthmatics. These medications could make it more difficult to manage diabetes.

Surgery

Graves' disease can also be treated with surgery to remove all or part of your thyroid (thyroidectomy or subtotal thyroidectomy). You'll probably require therapy following the procedure in order to give your body the normal dose of thyroid hormones.

The vocal cord nerve and the tiny glands (parathyroid glands) next to your thyroid gland may be damaged during this procedure, which increases the risk of complications. A hormone made by your parathyroid glands regulates the quantity of calcium in your blood. Under the supervision of a surgeon skilled in thyroid surgery, complications are uncommon. After this surgery, you will always need to take thyroid medication.

Treating the ophthalmopathy of Graves

Using over-the-counter artificial tears during the day and lubricating gels at night can help manage mild Graves' ophthalmopathy symptoms. Your doctor might suggest if your symptoms are more severe:

Corticosteroids

Corticosteroid therapy, such as prednisone, may reduce eyelid swelling. Fluid retention, weight gain, blood sugar and blood pressure elevations, as well as mood swings, are possible side effects.

Teprotumumab (Tepezza), a drug. This drug may be used to treat Graves' ophthalmopathy. Every three weeks, it is administered eight times via IV in the arm.

145

It may result in negative side effects like nausea, constipation, muscle spasms, and high blood sugar. As a relatively new drug, its function in treating Graves' opthalmopathy is still being established.

Prisms

Due to Graves' disease or as a result of the surgery to treat Graves' disease, you might experience double vision. Prisms in your glasses might be able to reduce your double vision, but they don't always work.

surgical procedure for decompression of the orbit. In this procedure, your surgeon removes the bone that connects your sinuses, the air spaces next to your orbit, and your eye socket (orbit). Your eyes now have space to return to their original position.

When pressure on the optic nerve threatens to cause vision loss, this treatment is typically used. Double vision is one of the potential issues.

Radiotherapy in orbit

Although the advantages are unclear, this was once a widely used treatment for this condition. Some of the tissue behind your eyes is destroyed using focused X-rays over the course of several days. If your eye issues worsen and corticosteroids alone aren't working or being tolerated well, your doctor may advise trying this.

Treatment for Graves' disease does not always result in improvements in Graves' ophthalmopathy. For three to six months, Graves' ophthalmopathy symptoms may even worsen. After that, Graves' ophthalmopathy signs and symptoms typically stabilize for about a year before starting to improve, frequently on their own.

Lifestyle and DIY treatments

Make your mental and physical health a top priority if you have Graves' disease:

- Maintaining a healthy diet and engaging in regular exercise can accelerate the resolution of some symptoms during treatment and improve your overall wellbeing. For instance, because your thyroid regulates your metabolism, you might find that after the hyperthyroidism is treated, you tend to put on weight. Weight-bearing exercises can help maintain bone density and prevent the brittle bones that can accompany Graves' disease.

- Stress can worsen or trigger Graves' disease, so reducing stress may be beneficial. You can unwind and improve your mood by walking, taking a warm bath, or listening to music. Develop a plan with your physician that incorporates a healthy diet, regular exercise, and downtime into your daily schedule.

because of Graves' ophthalmopathy.

If you have Graves' ophthalmopathy, these steps may help your eyes feel better:

- Your eyes should be treated with cool compresses. The additional moisture might calm your eyes.

- Put on sunglasses. Your eyes become more sensitive to bright light and more susceptible to UV rays when they protrude. Your eyes will experience less wind-induced irritability if you wear sunglasses that encircle your head on both sides.

- Make use of lubricating eyedrops. Your eyes may no longer feel dry and itchy if you use eyedrops. An overnight application of a paraffin-based gel is possible.

- Adjust your bed's headrest. By keeping your head higher than the rest of your body, you can reduce the buildup of fluid in your head and potentially relieve pressure on your eyes.

- No smoking. Graves' ophthalmopathy is made worse by smoking.
- regarding Graves' dermopathy.
- Use over-the-counter creams or ointments containing hydrocortisone to relieve swelling and reddening if the disease (Graves' dermopathy) affects your skin.
- Compression leg wraps could also be beneficial.

Graves disease treatment

In general, Graves' disease-related hyperthyroidism is easily managed, safely treated, and nearly always successfully treated. However, the majority of treatments for hyperthyroidism eventually lead to hypothyroidism or an underactive thyroid gland. With surgery or radioactive iodine use, this might happen sooner. 1-6.

Radioiodine treatment

In the United States, radioiodine therapy is the most widely used therapy for treating Graves' disease. The patient is given pills containing radioactive iodine-131 to take orally.

The thyroid gland selectively absorbs this radioactive I because it needs iodine to produce thyroid hormone. The radioactive Iodine used for thyroid scans is weaker than the I131. While leaving other tissues unaffected, it serves to gradually destroy the thyroid gland's cells.

When administered in high doses, can completely shut down the thyroid gland.

Some doctors opt for this.

However, some people prefer to use smaller doses to restore hormone production to a healthy level.

Multiple sessions of this therapy might be required. Results of the therapy frequently take time to manifest and can take weeks or even months to do so.

may make Graves' ophthalmopathy worse, according to some studies. To fully comprehend the risks, these patients may require consultation. To lessen these negative effects, they may require additional steroid medications.

Despite the fact that is not known to cause birth defects or infertility, it is generally not advised and should not be used in pregnant women due to the possibility of harm to the fetal thyroid gland.

Breastfeeding mothers should also avoid it.

Iodine that is radioactive can harm a developing fetus' thyroid and is transferred from mother to child through breast milk.

This treatment may eventually result in hypothyroidism or a thyroid gland that is underactive. Synthetic thyroid hormone is required as replacement therapy for hypothyroidism patients.

Graves' disease medications

Antithyroid drugs and beta blockers are two common medications for Graves' disease.

Drugs called beta blockers are used to treat high blood pressure. These medications as-is do not lessen thyroid hormone production, but they may ease anxiety symptoms like palpitations and fast heartbeat. They also alleviate tremor and shakiness symptoms.

Methimazole, propylthiouracil, and carbimazole are all antithyroid medications. These affect the thyroid gland and stop it from absorbing and using iodine, which is necessary for the production of thyroid hormones. Typically, the effects of these medications are only short-term and do not last.

Hormone levels must also be continuously monitored.

The pre-treatment of patients over the age of 60, women who are pregnant, nursing, or who have other health issues is best done with these medications before they decide to undergo radioiodine therapy.

Following radioiodine therapy, antithyropid medications may be used.

Women who are pregnant can only take propylthiouracil. They are unable to take methimazole because it can harm the fetal thyroid gland by crossing the placental barrier.

The smallest dose of either medication is advised for nursing mothers. Antithyroid medications frequently cause allergic reactions, rashes and itching, liver damage, a reduction in white blood cell production, an increased risk of infection, among other side effects.

Graves' disease and thyroid surgery
The least frequently chosen method for treating Graves' disease is thyroid surgery. Patients who are not candidates for radioactive iodine or antithyroid medications may opt for this alternative, though.

This includes those who are expecting, those who have thyroid cancer suspicions, and those who have not responded to other treatments. Thyroid cancer is not a consequence of Graves' disease.

The thyroid gland is partially or completely removed during surgery. To prevent a recurrence of hyperthyroidism, some doctors prefer to remove the entire thyroid gland. The patient must take thyroxine replacement therapy in the form of pills for the rest of their lives as this may cause hypothyroidism.

Additionally, there are risks associated with surgery, such as bleeding into the neck's major blood vessels and nerves, damage to the parathyroid glands, etc. The thyroid gland and the parathyroid glands are situated very close together. They aid in maintaining healthy blood calcium levels.

Graves' disease treatment for eye issues

With the aforementioned treatment, Graves' disease-related eye problems might not be alleviated. You might need to handle these differently. Eye drops are recommended to soothe dry and itchy eyes.

Prednisone and other steroid medications are occasionally prescribed to suppress immune response and offer comfort.

People who experience double vision, blurred vision, or other vision issues may require prescription lenses and glasses

To lessen eyelid swelling, doctors advise patients to sleep with their heads elevated. In order to avoid dry eyes at night, those who are unable to completely close their eyelids may use special taping.

The role of vitamins and minerals in the thyroid

We are all aware that eating the right foods will help us get all the vitamins and minerals we need to stay healthy. Thyroid deficiency can be brought on by a lack of specific vitamins and minerals, and if you have thyroid deficiency, the vitamins you are ingesting cannot be processed properly.

Nowadays, a lot of people have hectic schedules and little time for healthy eating. Without realizing it, a lot of young people skip meals in an effort to lose weight. This can have negative effects on the thyroid gland. Even if you try to eat healthfully, by the time we buy, prepare, and cook regular foods, most of the nutrients have vanished. Occasionally, supplements are necessary to maintain a healthy thyroid.

A vegetarian or vegan diet lacking in protein can also harm the thyroid. Nowadays, doctors are less likely to check you for vitamin and mineral deficiencies unless you visit an alternative therapist. You might be shocked to learn that many of these, particularly vitamin D and vitamin B12, are deficient in you. Pernicious anemia is becoming more prevalent, so the next time you visit your doctor, make sure you have these deficiencies checked out.

The following is a list of vitamins and minerals that are important for thyroid health.

1. A vitamin, not a carotenoid

An early form of vitamin A is carotene. No matter how many carrots you eat or other foods you consume, a hypothyroid gland cannot effectively convert carotene to usable vitamin A. You eating won't make a difference. Vitamin A needs protein in order to be absorbed by the body, so if you consume little protein, you may not get enough of this vitamin. Your capacity to produce TSH is constrained if you are deficient in vitamin A. The body needs this vitamin to change T4 into T3. Try taking vitamin A supplements along with more protein to see if it helps if you find that the lights are too bright or night driving is a problem.

2. B complex vitamin

Although each B vitamin plays a distinct role, they are all essential for healthy thyroid function.

3. Thiamine (BL)

If your thyroid is overactive, you urgently need this vitamin.

4. Riboflavin, vitamin B2

Because the thyroid and adrenal glands are unable to secrete hormones, thyroid function is suppressed when vitamin B2 levels are low.

5. Niacin, B3

This is required to maintain the health and effectiveness of all the body's cells, including the endocrine glands.

6. Pyridoxine, also known as vitamin B6

The thyroid cannot effectively produce hormones from its iodine raw material without this vitamin. An overactive thyroid requires more pyridoxine B6. People with an overactive thyroid and those who are B6 deficient frequently experience weakness of the muscles.

7. B12

Vitamin B12 cannot be absorbed by those with underactive or absent thyroids. Mental illness, different neurological disorders, neuralgia, neuritis, and bursitis can all result from a severe B12 deficiency. The "normal range" of B12, according to some doctors, should be at least 500 - 1,300 pg/ml (rather than 200 - 1,100).

8. The vitamin C

For optimal health, the thyroid gland requires vitamin C. The thyroid gland secretes too much hormone when there has been a prolonged deficiency. Vitamin C is actually drained from the tissues in the bodies of people with an overactive thyroid, so they require extra vitamin C.

9. Supplement D

It has been discovered that taking vitamin D prevents the typical rapid excretion of calcium in people with an overactive thyroid, thereby preventing osteoporosis.

10.   E vitamin

A higher intake of this vitamin is frequently required by individuals with an overactive thyroid to counteract the significant amounts of the vitamin depleted from the system, as vitamin E deficiency encourages the thyroid gland to secrete too much hormone as well as too little TSH by the pituitary gland.

11.   Calcium

The amount of calcium we get from dairy products is often too low. This is crucial to prevent bone loss, especially in those who are overactive.

12.   Magnesium

Magnesium should be supplemented because it's necessary for the transformation of T4 into T3. Magnesium loss through urination can be very rapid for some people. Additionally, it appears that a diet heavy in caffeine and refined foods will promote magnesium loss.

13.   Selenium

The enzyme in the body that changes T4 to T3 relies heavily on selenium. Without it, T3 cannot be produced in the required quantities, and even when blood test levels are normal, organs will behave hypothyroidally.

14.   Zinc

Studies have demonstrated that a zinc deficiency is a side effect of both hypo- and hyperthyroidism. Additionally, it affects how well the immune system functions. Obese people have been shown to have low zinc levels. This mineral is essential because it helps turn T4 into T3.

In spite of having high levels, Dr. Arem advises taking supplements if you are overactive. When your levels are normal or close to normal, he believes it is safer to begin taking them if you have hypothyroidism. He explains that taking iron at the same time as thyroid hormone will cause some of the thyroid hormone to bind with the iron and prevent the absorption of the thyroid hormone. Thyroid hormone absorption may be affected if fiber and calcium carbonate are taken at the same time.

How does stress impact the body?

Hormone levels fluctuate when the body is subjected to stress, whether it be physical, mental, or life-threatening events. The hormones cortisol, insulin, prolactin, and thyroid hormones are just a few of the ones the body's many hormones that are impacted by stress. Everybody experiences this "fight or flight" response, which causes their hormone levels to change.

Stress is not always bad, despite the common perception that it is. Positive life events, such as starting a new job or having a baby, can occasionally cause stress.

When someone is experiencing chronic stress, it becomes a problem. Certain endocrine and autoimmune disorders have been linked to a sustained state of stress. Additionally, stress has been shown to exacerbate the symptoms of pre-existing disorders and to start new ones.

What is the effect of stress on TED?

Long-term stress can cause thyroid hormones to go into overdrive. This may result in a number of endocrine disorders, including Graves' disease. Hyperthyroidism is a result of this autoimmune condition, which causes the thyroid to produce too much hormone.

A frequent side effect of Graves' disease is TED. Up to half of people with Graves' disease are affected by it because it is so widespread. In cases of hyperthyroidism, TED occurs in about 90% of cases.

Stress can cause a previously inactive state to become active in people who have already been diagnosed with TED. eye inflammation and redness.

- eyelid swelling.

171

- Diplopia is the medical term for double vision.

- eyeball protrusion or bulging (proptosis).

There is some evidence that stress can exacerbate symptoms and exacerbate active TED.

TED patients' stress-reduction recommendations.

While medications and other treatments can aid in managing TED symptoms, lowering stress levels can also be beneficial.

The following suggestions and methods can help you manage stress:

Adopt a nutritious, well-balanced diet

Consider a diet rich in lean protein, fruits, and vegetables.

Regularly moving around

A great way to reduce stress is to exercise. Feel-good endorphins are produced during aerobic exercise like walking, jogging, and swimming, which can help reduce stress.

Put an end to your smoking. Compared to non-smokers, smokers have a 7 times higher risk of developing TED and a 2x higher risk of Graves' disease.

Utilize breathing exercises to relax. Yoga, meditation, and deep breathing are a few examples of these.

Spend time relaxing by gardening, listening to music, being in nature, and spending time with loved ones.

By altering your hormone levels, stress can make TED symptoms worse. Try the aforementioned advice to lessen stress in your life, especially if you've discovered that TED symptoms are brought on by high levels of stress. Consider discussing healthy coping strategies for stressful life events and situations with your doctor.

www.ingramcontent.com/pod-product-compliance
Lightning Source LLC
Chambersburg PA
CBHW050811260726
48660CB00004B/1371